The New
Self Help Series
BODY ODOUR

The New Self Help Series
BODY ODOUR

LEON CHAITOW
N.D., D.O.

Thorsons
An Imprint of HarperCollinsPublishers

Thorsons
An Imprint of HarperCollins*Publishers*
77–85 Fulham Palace Road,
Hammersmith, London W6 8JB

Published by Thorsons 1994
10 9 8 7 6 5 4 3 2 1

A catalogue record for this book
is available from the British Library

ISBN 0 7225 2954 6

Typeset by Harper Phototypesetters Limited
Northampton, England

Printed in Great Britain by
HarperCollinsManufacturing Glasgow

Contents

Note to reader

Before following the self-help advice given in
this book, readers are earnestly urged to give
careful consideration to the nature of their
particular health problem, and to consult a
competent physician if in any doubt. This
book should not be regarded as a substitute
for professional medical treatment, and
whilst every care is taken to ensure the
accuracy of the content, the author and
publishers cannot accept legal responsibility
for any problem arising out of the experi-
mentation with the methods described.

CHAPTER ONE

Body Odour – Why Does it Happen?

B.O. – body odour – has become a major industry – or rather the suppression of B.O. is now big business. Products that address this problem (or imagined problem for many people) now dominate entire aisles of supermarkets and hordes of people are involved in manufacturing, marketing and advertising them. There used to be an advertisement for a popular brand of soap with a caption telling us that this was the product to use for the problem about which 'your best friends won't tell you'. We seem to have moved beyond soap, with deodorants and antiperspirants, not to mention perfumes for men and women, now selling themselves as the means to mask or prevent that unspeakable problem that your best friends are likely to remain silent about.

Certainly we all 'smell' to some extent – otherwise dogs would have trouble recognising us.

However, our own sense of smell is somewhat less efficient than the canine variety and so, for most people, body odour has to be pretty pungent to be upsetting.

There are of course degrees of offensiveness in body odour – and what one person may find thoroughly unpleasant someone else might not mind, and others might actually like. The recent biography of Albert Einstein reports that his interest in women was greater 'the more they smelled'. The reason for this is not as odd as it appears, since sweat carries in it minute substances called pheromones, which are important in signalling sexual interest inducing subconscious attraction in the opposite sex. Researchers at Warwick University in the UK claim to have identified 50 chemicals that make up human sex-pheromones, found in sweat produced by the glands on the face, underarms and genitals.

Despite some of the chemicals in sweat being 'attractive' in this way, the truth is that some people do seem to carry a particularly offensive odour. Unpleasant body odour can cause enormous distress to the person affected, sometimes leading to the need for counselling and psychological help. In a recent medical research study it was found that many people with B.O. reported problems with relationships, wrecked promotion prospects at work, educational underachievement because of teasing and bullying, stress leading to alcoholism or excessive tobacco or drug use, as well as feelings of shame, embarrassment, low self-esteem, isolation, frustration, anxiety and depression. It is also not uncommon for a person with B.O. to be completely unaware of the problem.

The causes of unpleasant body odour are many and varied. Let's take a look at the most likely offenders.

HYGIENE

The commonest cause of B.O. is careless hygiene relating to bathing and the cleaning of clothes. When sweat produced by our 2 to 3 million sweat glands is left on the surface of the body (or on our clothes) for a number of hours, it is acted upon by bacteria that *can* produce an odour. If sweat is not washed off the body or clothes, bacterial action will created a smell, and this smell is more likely to be offensive if someone sweats excessively.

HEALTH IMBALANCES

Sweat and bacterial action therefore account for some people's problem, but they are not the whole story. Many people in, for example, a particular working environment are under the same conditions of atmospheric humidity and heat, performing similar functions in terms of physical activity, and are sweating to a similar degree – and yet only some will produce strong body odours.

Another important factor is each individual's internal biochemistry, and this can be affected by a deficiency of various substances such as digestive enzymes, vitamins and minerals, and also by toxicity and related health problems. Because of these individual biochemical differences some people will literally reek of particular spices and herbs (garlic, for example) if they were eaten the previous day, whereas others (the majority) will not be much affected whatever they eat.

Detoxification is a process that is taking place in our bodies all the time, as they work to eliminate the toxins and other undesirable substances in our food, drink and environments, along with the natural waste products of bodily function. The efficiency or otherwise of your internal detoxification processes is therefore important in determining whether you have B.O.

Your body's ability to process toxins and other waste materials is in turn affected by other imbalances. The vital mineral zinc, for example, is known to be deficient in many people with B.O. Zinc takes part in many important body processes involving detoxification, and a deficiency of it seems to not only to contribute to B.O., but also leads to a less efficient sense of smell – so the person whose B.O. results from zinc deficiency will also be less likely to be aware of the fact themselves.

Medical tests at Imperial College in London have shown that some people with B.O. have imbalances affecting the 'friendly bacteria' that live inside all of our digestive systems. This can lead to aggravation of B.O.

B.O. can be associated with a number of health problems, including liver dysfunction, diabetes, digestive problems (parasites etc.) and yeast infections. Some people with yeast conditions carry a 'beer' smell, since yeast can turn sugar into alcohol very rapidly.

STRESS

Stress often dramatically increases body odour, and in order to understand how this happens we need to take a look at the nervous system, since it controls the degree of sweating that takes place.

The autonomic nervous system, which takes care of the body functions that are outside our direct influence, is divided into two parts: the sympathetic and the parasympathetic. In some people (the excitable greyhound/racehorse types) the sympathetic aspect of the nervous system is dominant, whereas in others (the calm bulldog/ carthorse type) the parasympathetic aspect dominates. Someone whose sympathetic nervous system is easily aroused, startled or upset will sweat more than someone whose parasympathetic nervous system is more dominant and who is therefore more phlegmatic and apparently unemotional. Heightened sympathetic activity therefore encourages the tendency to B.O. through

5

increased sweating and subsequent bacterial action.

Fortunately we can influence our autonomic nervous system by using a number of techniques which increase the relaxation potential, produce calming effects and which reduce our levels of easy arousal by stress.

INHERITED FACTORS

There is medical evidence that some forms of unpleasant body odour are inherited, so that if one member of a family is affected there are likely to be others with similar problems. In these instances certain foods are not completely digested and broken down because of inherited enzyme deficiencies, or acquired digestive problems, leading to a particular body odour in which a strong 'fishy' smell is noted. This is particularly likely to occur around period time or when the contraceptive pill is being used. Dietary changes, particularly reducing foods rich in lysine and lecithin (see chapter 5), seem to be able to reduce the intensity of the problem in many cases.

WHAT'S TO BE DONE?

One option is to cover up the problem – disguising the B.O. – which is a reasonable approach as long as the underlying causes are also being dealt with and, most importantly, if the 'cover-up' method does not in itself produce new health problems. The 'first aid' suggestions in this book involve natural products that do not have the same negative side-effects as many commercial products used in the deodorant industry, largely through their use of aluminium salts and the potential dangers of excessive use of that substance.

Another option is to take care of some pretty basic hygienic considerations, which should clear away the worst of the problem.

We can also look at areas of health that affect B.O., including the liver and digestive system, as well as some specific infections (Candida albicans yeast infection for example) and can consider some self-help methods for detoxification and regeneration to improve these aspects of our health.

The possibility of nutritional deficiency needs to be looked at seriously, since this is probably the most common cause of body odour apart from hygiene.

Finally, we can monitor our levels of stress and the response of our nervous system to that stress, and if necessary we can introduce simple exercises in relaxation which can profoundly change levels of arousal and stress. We can also make some specific adjustments to our lifestyle and habits which can significantly improve any imbalance in the autonomic nervous system.

The next chapter looks at the many possible and

sometimes interacting causes of B.O., after which a selection of self-help measures are presented from which you can choose. One way or another we should be able to get B.O. under control.

CHAPTER TWO

Why Some People Sweat More Than Others

We sweat mainly in order to control our body's temperature – as the sweat evaporates we get cooler, a process that is more efficient in a dry than a humid atmosphere. We can lose pints of liquid per hour if it is hot enough. In air-conditioned or less humid situations we continue to perspire but usually don't notice it as much because of the evaporation of the sweat.

The sweat itself consists mainly of water and salt (sodium chloride) but there are also certain levels of fat and protein present when it leaves the more specialised pores under the arms, on the hands and on the soles of our feet. These ingredients (salt, fats and proteins) provide the basic smell of sweat. Since the levels of protein and fat vary from person to person, as well as from race to race, so (slightly) does the characteristic odour vary. Under normal health conditions fresh sweat does not produce the odour of B.O. This develops only after the bacteria that live on our skin surface have had a chance to act on the sweat for at least a couple of hours.

We can see therefore that the secondary function of perspiring is to act as a channel of elimination and excretion – when the body needs to do so it can load additional material into the sweat to get it out of the body. If the sweat carries large amounts of toxic debris from the body this can produce specific unpleasant odours.

WHAT INFLUENCES SWEAT PRODUCTION?

Temperature

When the atmospheric temperature is high we will sweat more, and if the humidity of the air (how much liquid it carries) is high we will notice sweating more because evaporation is not efficient when the air has a lot of liquid in it – the sweat stays on the skin surface and becomes obvious. Surprisingly, perhaps, we sweat quite a lot even on a cold day – about half a litre of liquid.

Stress

If the sympathetic nervous system is overactive we perspire more, and this is more likely to happen when we are nervous, upset or anxious – hence the expression 'sweating with fear'. Our emotional state is therefore directly connected to our sweat levels and so you can often influence chronic excessive sweating problems through stress reduction approaches.

Medications and Stimulants

Some medications can make us sweat more – aspirin, for example, and, less obviously, tea, coffee and alcohol. The use of stimulants of this sort needs to be considered as a cause of excessive sweating in some people.

Blood Sugar

When blood sugar levels are low we break into a sweat ('cold sweat') because one of the hormonal centres that controls our levels of sugar, the adrenal glands, becomes active and this stimulates the part of the brain that makes us sweat. If you have ever missed a meal and developed a sinking, fainting feeling you will know exactly what this is like.

Hormonal Imbalances

Other hormonal activity, such as a thyroid gland that is overproducing its secretions, will increase our metabolic rate (our internal level of function and heat production) and will therefore encourage more sweating. There are simple home tests to evaluate whether this is likely to be a factor in any given case.

Periods of our life when hormonal imbalances and changes occur – such as puberty and menopause – are likely also to be periods when sweat production is more erratic, and this can cause perspiration to be greatly overproduced, as with 'hot flushes'. There are a number of natural ways of providing help during these periods of transition.

Finally, some people just produce more sweat than others for no obvious reason. Medically this is called 'essential hidrosis'.

WHAT CAN WE DO ABOUT EXCESSIVE SWEATING?

A variety of more natural methods of camouflaging natural odours are available than those offered by commercial anti-perspirants and deodorants, many of which contain highly undesirable levels of aluminium. These methods are outlined in chapter 3.

As hard as we try we can influence the atmosphere around us only to a limited extent. However, by diligent use of adequate ventilation, control of air movement, ionisers and humidifiers – and by controlling internal temperature levels as much as possible – it is possible to minimise the worst aspects of some modern buildings, which encourage B.O. through their construction and design. Some suggestions for creating an ideal work and living environment are given in chapter 10.

Control of what is eliminated in our sweat is also possible to a degree by careful evaluation of our levels of toxicity followed by appropriate nutritional action, and by encouraging skin activity towards a more normal function using a variety of simple techniques. Directions and suggestions are given in chapter 6.

Specific action to reduce levels of arousal, involving breathing and relaxation techniques, can lesson the tendency for sympathetic nervous system overactivity. Suggestions are given in chapter 4.

Thyroid and other hormonal imbalances can be helped by nutritional and herbal methods and advice on these approaches is given in chapter 9.

There is also specific consideration of the importance of zinc deficiency in B.O. See chapter 8, which deals with general nutrition.

By tackling first aid as well as long-term strategies to improve internal and external factors relating to body odour problems, a programme should emerge that anyone can apply at home. Appropriate expert help may be needed where self-help measures are not desirable or indicated.

CHAPTER THREE

First Aid for Body Odour

Cleanliness is the first and major priority if B.O. is to be avoided, so why not use commercial soaps, antiperspirants and deodorants? There are several good reasons.

Antibacterial or germicidal soaps, possibly containing hexachlorophene, might be useful in the short term, but because they also eliminate or weaken the normal bacterial inhabitants of our skin and are potentially toxic, they can produce more problems than they solve. Not all bacteria are harmful – in fact we have an important symbiotic relationship with many that live in and on us. Antibacterial soap can reduce their efficiency, which leaves us susceptible to fungal growth on the skin. It's not a good idea to wash these friendly bacteria off.

Most commercial soaps are alkaline and this reduces the natural acidity of the skin, causing increased activity of less friendly bacteria. So only acidic soaps which encourage normal bacterial activity should be used.

Deodorants and antiperspirants containing aluminium – which means most commercial versions – are worrying because of the possibility that the aluminium in them could be absorbed through the skin and find its way to the brain. Aluminium is implicated in Alzheimer's Disease – and exchanging body odour for holes in the brain would not seem to be a good bargain.

SAFE STRATEGIES FOR BODY ODOUR

Clothing

Clothes worn next to the skin must be fresh on each day and must have been thoroughly washed and aired since the previous wearing. Vests, underwear, blouses and shirts, as well as socks and stockings, all need to be worn only when freshly washed and aired. All too often body odour is really 'clothes odour' resulting from bacterial action on stale sweat that has impregnated the clothes.

Wear only natural fibre underwear such as cotton, linen or silk, since artificial fibres prevent normal skin functions and reduce the presence of oxygen, which encourages bacterial activity on sweat. Try also to wear loose fitting clothing so that air can circulate, allowing sweat to evaporate more normally than constricting clothing does.

Baths and Showers

Take a bath at night and a shower in the morning. Wash the feet, underarms and body surface using an appropriate soap (see below for suggestions). If you use normal commercial (alkaline soaps) you will almost certainly make body odour worse by damaging the natural acidic controls over bacterial activity.

A variety of aromatherapy oils can be used in the bath, which will leave a lingering pleasant perfume and produce general health benefits. Among those suggested for people with body odour problems are basil, chamomile, cypress, lavender, neroli, rose, sandalwood, sage and vetiver. See pages 74–78 for details about how to use aromatherapy oils when bathing.

For sweaty feet use a few drops of cypress oil rubbed onto the soles of the feet and between the toes every day until the problem improves.

Soaps

Several slightly acidic soaps are available which are particularly suited to people with body odour tendencies. They include a cleansing bar made from Austrian Moor, a peat-like substance that contains hundreds of medicinal plants and is widely used for health and beauty products. This unperfumed cleansing bar provides the essential slightly acid effect that keeps the skin healthy.

Dead Sea mud soap from Israel is highly recommended for body odour and skin problems, as is the foot care cream which retards excessive sweating of the feet as well as having beneficial effects on the skin of the area.

French clay also makes a good soap, because clay has a powerful attraction to toxic materials and odours. Look out also for body scrubs made from natural substances like rice bran. These are invigorating and also remove dead skin.

Deodorants

After every bath or shower gently rub the skin with a deodorant stone or crystal. These natural mineral salt 'stones' were developed in Thailand over 100 years ago and are now widely available from health stores and some pharmacies. They consist of a solid, crystal-like stone made of potassium sulphate derived from certain volcanic regions. The small amount of potassium sulphate that adheres to the skin when it is rubbed on the wet body has an antibacterial effect, and because it has a large molecular structure it is not absorbed through the skin. *The film of potassium sulphate has a slight acidic effect on the skin*, which it needs after a wash, and this non-sticky shield lasts for up to 24 hours, preventing bacterial activity and so retarding B.O. (even under the arm).

There are no allergic problems with these stones, and they contain none of the aluminium salts that are present in commercial deodorants. Used daily these crystals should last at least a year and often up to two years.

There are also a number of deodorants available that do not have an antiperspirant effect and do not contain aluminium salts. Look for them in health stores and pharmacies.

As an alternative to commercial deodorants, sprinkling baking soda (bicarbonate of soda) between the toes and in the armpits is an effective and safe method.

Homoeopathy

Homoeopathic medicines are available through many pharmacies and health stores. The following are recommended for body odour problems:

Hepar Sulph 6C – if there is profuse sweating
    and the skin is sensitive to the touch
Merc. Sol 6C – if perspiration is offensive and/or
    stains the clothes yellow
Sulphur 6C – if skin looks unhealthy and if the
    feet are particularly a problem with odour
Thuja 6C – if sweating occurs particularly on
    parts of the body that are not covered.

Nutritional Supplements

Every day take 30 milligrams of chelated zinc and 100 milligrams of vitamin B6 (see chapter 8 for more details). By taking care of what you wear, by regular bathing and showering with appropriate soaps, by use of natural antiperspirants and deodorants, and the employment of homoeopathic first aid as appropriate and the regular supplementation of important nutrients, you have every chance of reducing B.O. dramatically.

If B.O. is associated with more complex problems, as outlined in the opening chapters of the book, then read on for practical self-help advice.

CHAPTER FOUR

The Link between Stress, Arousal and Sweating

The more anxious you are the more easily aroused you will be and – since increased arousal stimulates the sympathetic nervous system, which controls your sweat activity – the more you will tend to sweat. Because of that, any body odour problem you have will be accentuated. The less anxious you are, the less aroused you will be, the less dominant your sympathetic nervous system will be and the less you will tend to sweat.

There are a number of ways that doctors can assess your arousal, including measurement of the electrical resistance of your skin or the amount of activity in key muscles when you are resting or the type of brain-wave most commonly active in your brain. If you want to test yourself, you can easily recognise that your arousal levels are high when you develop any of the following signs:

- being more restless and/or easily upset than usual
- difficulty in relaxing

- a disturbed sleep pattern
- sighing a lot or breathing more shallowly than usual
- difficulty in concentrating
- feeling on edge
- an almost constant sense of anxiety.

HOW RELAXED ARE YOU?

There is a simple formula that you can look at to decide whether you are taking account all of the needs that might be influencing your ability to cope with stress. If you are to be really relaxed and able to cope with stress:

- Your diet needs to meet your requirements while your intake of 'tasty toxins' and stimulants needs to be as low as possible.
- Your muscles need to release their tensions, leading to a saving in wasted energy. This might call for massage, stretching exercises, hydrotherapy or better nutrition. Muscular release is the first step towards calming your mind, since your mind cannot be calm if your muscles are in tension.
- Your breathing needs to be full and free. Massage, exercise, stretching, hydrotherapy with essential oils and specific breathing exercises can all help this. This leads to better circulation and oxygenation and has specific effects on feelings of anxiety and being 'stressed out', as the body and mind cannot relax or cope well with stress if they are poorly supplied with vital oxygen and nutrients by a good blood supply.

- Once you have achieved muscular release and full breathing your mind needs to be able to stay still and focused and to release itself from the chatter of daily events and anxieties. This leads to a profound sense of being centred and at ease – and it shows to those around you as your ability to concentrate and remember details is boosted and your whole being reflects calmness.
- And finally, once you have taken care of your muscular and breathing requirements and your mind is still, you need to exercise it in creative visualisation.

To summarise – muscular release, full breathing, mental calm and guided imagery, *in this sequence*, can protect you from the worst effects of stress as well as allowing you to feel and function and look at your best, with energy to spare. These simple steps reduce overarousal of the sympathetic nervous system and cut down tendencies to sweat inappropriately.

If being aroused and sweating more than is called for by virtue of your physical activity shows that you are anxious, you can learn to reduce your anxiety level. You may find this surprisingly easy. You can start from a number of different places in order to achieve this, all will lead to the same result if successful – a reduction in anxiety and in all probability a reduction in the rate of perspiration. The following exercises in breathing, relaxation and visualisation show you how.

BREATHING

There are many exercises to help improve breathing but there is just one that has been shown in medical studies effectively to reduce arousal and anxiety levels . This is an exercise based on traditional yoga methods of breathing. The pattern is as follows:

1 Having placed yourself in a comfortable (ideally seated) position you inhale *fully* while silently counting up to no more than three (ideally two). Translated into practical terms this means that you fill your lungs fairly quickly. The counting is necessary because the timing of the inhalation and exhalation phase of breathing is critical in this exercise.

2 Without pausing to hold your breath at all you then exhale *fully* taking four, five or six seconds to do so, again counting silently at the same speed as when you inhaled.

3 Repeat the inhalation for two seconds and the exhalation – the objective is that in time, with practice, you should make this exhalation phase last eight seconds.

4 All inhalation is through the nose if possible, while exhalation can be through the nose or mouth. Most importantly the breathing out must be slow and continuous. It is no use breathing the air out in two seconds and then simply waiting until the count reaches five or six before inhaling again.

5 Repeat the cycles of inhalation and exhalation

for several minutes with at least six cycles per minutes. Each cycle should eventually last ten seconds, two in and eight out, although at first you may find that two in and three or four out is all you can manage. By the time you have completed 10 or so cycles your sense of anxiety should be much reduced and your awareness of pain less.

6 Do this exercise for a few minutes every hour *if you are anxious or whenever stress seem to be increasing*.

Focus on Breathing Muscles

Before doing the exercise described above sit or stand in front of a mirror and observe your shoulders as you breathe deeply. Do they rise towards your ears as you inhale? If so you are using certain muscles that attach to neck and shoulders as well as the upper ribs in a way that should only happen when you are or have been running. To use them when seated or standing shows they are overworking and this will influence your breathing mechanics in a negative way.

To retrain yourself out of this habit, which is all it is, and help reduce the tendency it produces to hyperventilate (and therefore increase anxiety/arousal levels) you should do the following exercise, either separately from the one above or as part of it.

1 Sit in a chair that has arms and rest your arms on the chair.

2 As you practise deep breathing make sure that
your elbows are firmly pressed downwards
towards the floor, against the arms of the
chair, and that your abdomen moves forward.
This guarantees that the diaphragm is working
normally.

That is all there is to the exercise, since while you
are pressing down with your elbows it is impossible
to use the muscles that you were previously using,
and you are obliged to use the correct breathing
muscles. Do this at the same time as the rhythmic
breathing described above or at another time until
you can sit in front of a mirror and inhale without
your shoulders lifting towards your ears.

RELAXATION

There are a vast number of relaxation exercises but
one in particular is quite suitable for self-treatment.
Other forms of relaxation are encouraged, since
anything that produces a reduction of muscular
tension and mental anxiety can only help reduce a
tendency to sweating.

Modified Autogenic Training

Autogenic training is best learned from a fully
trained instructor. However, the following modified
form is an excellent way of achieving some degree

of control over muscle tone and/or circulation, and therefore over stress.

1 Lie on the floor or bed in a comfortable position, with a small cushion under your head perhaps and with your knees bent if that makes your back feel easier. Have your eyes closed.

2 Focus your attention on your right hand or arm and silently say to yourself, 'my right arm (or hand) feels heavy'. Try to see your arm relaxed and heavy, its weight sinking into the surface it is resting on. Feel its weight. Over a period of about a minute repeat the affirmation as to its heaviness several times and try to stay focused on the weight and heaviness of the hand/arm. You will almost certainly lose focus as your attention wanders from time to time. This is part of the training in the exercise – to stay focused – so don't feel angry, just go back to your arm and its heaviness. You may or may not be able to sense the heaviness – it doesn't matter too much at first. If you do, stay with it and enjoy the sense of release, of letting go, that comes with it.

3 Next focus on your left hand/arm and do exactly the same thing for about a minute.

4 Move to your left leg and then your right leg, with similar timing, messages and focused attention.

5 Go back to your hand/arm and affirm a message that tells you that you sense a greater degree of warmth there: 'My hand is feeling warm (or hot).'

6 After a minute or so go to your left hand/arm, your left leg and then finally your right leg, each time with the warming message and attention. If warmth is sensed stay with it for a while and feel it spread. Enjoy it.

7 Finally, focus on your forehead and affirm that it feels cool and refreshed. Stay with this cool and calm thought for a minute before completing the exercise.

By repeating the whole exercise at least once a day (10 or 15 minutes is all it will take) you will gradually find you can stay focused on each region and sensation. 'Heaviness' represents what you feel when muscles relax and 'warmth' is what you feel when your circulation to an area is increased, while 'coolness' is the opposite, a reduction in circulation for a short while, which can be beneficial for your forehead region.

VISUALISATION

Visualisation is part of a programme that follows on from deep relaxation and asks you to use mental pictures in which harmonious, uplifting and safe images (a flowery sunlit meadow by a sparkling river; or a quiet beach scene; or a favourite garden or room, for example) are used to produce a profound state of contentment. The next state is to employ the mind to encourage healing of one sort or another, as in the examples above. Once imagination has been cultivated in this way you can become extremely creative.

People have altered and improved their health in many ways using these methods, by visualising changes taking place in comic-strip-like images. When you are deeply relaxed, for example, you can visualise yourself cool and content, using the sense of coolness you enjoyed in the final part of the autogenic training exercise as your model. You could see yourself in a snowy setting, or relaxed and walking slowly on a frosty lawn, or any other image that counteracts a feeling of being hot and bothered.

Whatever visualisation image you construct it is absolutely essential that relaxation be achieved first.

DEEP RELAXATION THROUGH WATER THERAPY

A final method for deep relaxation uses hydrotherapy, or water therapy. This method is called the Neutral Bath – neutral in that water is at the same temperature as your body. When you place yourself in a neutral bath a profoundly relaxing influence on the nervous system occurs. This was the main method of calming violent and disturbed patients in mental asylums before tranquillisers appeared!

A neutral bath is useful in all cases of anxiety, feelings of being stressed and for relieving chronic pain and/or insomnia. It is also a general tonic for the heart. It should not be used if you have a skin condition that reacts badly to water or if you have serious cardiac disease. (It may help, but get professional advice first.)

MATERIALS
All you need is a bathtub, water and a bath thermometer.

METHOD
Run a bath as full as possible and with the water as close to 97 F (36.1°C) as possible, and certainly not exceeding that temperature. The bath has its effect by being as close to body temperature as possible. Immersion in water at this neutral temperature has a profoundly relaxing, sedating effect and a calming influence on nervous system activity. Get into the bath so that, if possible, the water covers your shoulders, and support your head on a towel or sponge.

The thermometer should be in the bath and the temperature should not be allowed to drop below

92°F/33.3°C. It can be topped up periodically but must not exceed that 97°F/36.1°C limit. The duration of bath should be anything from 30 minutes to four hours – the longer the better as far as relaxation effects are concerned. After the bath pat yourself dry quickly and get into bed for at least an hour.

CHAPTER FIVE

Nutritional and Natural Self-Help Measures

There are some common health problems that can cause B.O. They include Candida, bowel parasites, constipation and low blood sugar, and a relatively rare condition known as fish-odour syndrome. This chapter looks at some safe and effective treatments for these conditions.

NOTE

If any of these conditions are present they should be dealt with before attempting the detoxification programme outlined in the next chapter.

CANDIDA

Candida is a chronic yeast infection that can cause a wide range of physical and emotional symptoms, and is a common cause of changes in digestive and other bodily functions which can contribute to or be the main cause of body odour. The subject deserves our special consideration. I have had many patients who, on entering my consulting room, brought with them an odour best described as 'beery'. That alcohol/yeasty smell derives from both the breath and the body, as it literally oozes from the pores. What is happening in these people's intestines has been described in the medical press as 'auto-brewery syndrome' – as yeast literally turns sugar into alcohol in the person's bowels.

There seems to be a rising tide of yeast infection problems, especially in women but not uncommonly in men as well. Women are more likely to be affected because of hormonal fluctuations that encourage yeast activity, and because of the widespread use of contraceptive medication (the Pill), which further encourages yeast to become active. An underlying influence on both sexes is the use of antibiotics, which damage the friendly bacteria in the bowel which are the main control factor that prevents yeast from spreading into the bowel when we are healthy. These factors together with a high-sugar diet – a modern phenomenon – seem to be the key reasons for the sudden explosion of candida-related health problems.

The most obvious aspects of yeast disease are seen in thrush eruptions in the mouth, throat, and vaginal area, but a huge range of other, apparently unrelated symptoms have been found to derive from candida activity in some people. These range from digestive upsets such as heartburn, diarrhoea and chronic bloating, to cystitis, skin eruptions, allergies, menstrual problems, constipation, anxiety, irritability and depression.

A systemic approach to such conditions – as opposed to simply treating the local outbreak of infection – will get the best results because these local outbreaks are *always* associated with a widespread reservoir of yeast in the intestinal tract, and until this is controlled the yeast will continue its activities.

Do you have a candida problem? The following questionnaires will help you identify whether yeast is part of your problem.

Drug Use History

1 Have you undergone a course of antibiotic treatment which lasted for eight weeks or longer or for shorter periods four or more times in one year?

2 Have you ever undergone a course in antibiotics for acne treatment for more than a month?

3 Have you been treated with steroid medication (cortisone, prednisone, etc.)?

4 Have you been on 'the Pill' for a year or more?

5 Have you received treatment with immune-suppressant medication?

6 Have you been pregnant more than once?

Symptom History

1 Have you had recurrent or persistent cystitis, vaginitis or prostatitis?
2 Do you have a history of endometriosis?
3 Have you had thrush (in the mouth or vagina) more than once?
4 Are you subject to athlete's foot or fungal problems with your nails or skin?
5 Do you suffer from a variety of allergies?
6 Are any of your symptoms worse after eating sugary foods or yeast-based foods or after being exposed to chemical smells?
7 Do you suffer from abdominal bloating regularly, or frequent diarrhoea or constipation?
8 Do you suffer from premenstrual symptoms such as fluid retention?
9 Do you suffer from lethargy, exhaustion, fatigue?
10 Do you crave sweet foods or alcohol?
11 Do your muscles ache or feel tingly or numb for no reason?
12 Do you suffer from impotence or lack of sexual drive?

If one or more of the questions in the first section are answered YES and two or more in the second section are answered YES then you are probably suffering from yeast-related ill-health and it could be playing a major part in any body odour problems you have.

The following is a summary of the best way of starting to control yeast.

Firstly it is necessary to understand that when Candida (thrush) affects the mouth or throat it is already widely spread in the intestines and possibly the vaginal area. This is why symptoms such as digestive distress (bloating, 'acid' stomach, diarrhoea or constipation) and genito-urinary problems (recurrent cystitis, vaginitis, etc.) are all too common along with mouth and throat infection by yeast. Any local treatment focusing only on the mouth (or vagina) will have limited short-term effects, so it is necessary to pay particular attention to the main colonies of yeast which will be flourishing in the bowel.

Everyone has some Candida but it is usually controlled efficiently by the immune system and by huge colonies of friendly bacteria living in our intestinal tract (including the mouth, which is the start of the intestinal tract) and on our skin. Yeast often gets out of hand, though, when antibiotics (which damage the friendly bacteria) and other medication are used too enthusiastically or too often – especially if the diet is unbalanced, with too much sugar and not enough nutrient-rich foods.

An approach that uses a *triple attack* is usually best in order to avoid a repetitive cycle in which Candida outbreaks occur whenever you are under stress or your immune system is under pressure (with another infection, for example). The threefold approach is as follows:

- Start to kill the yeast using a variety of herbal products such as garlic, caprylic acid (coconut plant extract), aloe vera juice and sometimes also the herbs hydrastis and echinacea (not for pregnant women).
- At the same time start to replenish the bowel flora using proven viable colonising strains of the friendly bacteria that usually inhabit the intestines: Lactobacillus acidophilus for the mouth, vagina and small intestine, and Bifidobacteria for the large intestine. These are the normal controlling element for Candida which are usually damaged when antibiotics or steroid drugs (including the Pill) are used medically, allowing the yeast to get out of hand.
- In addition a low-sugar/high-complex-carbohydrate diet is suggested, together with cultured (live) dairy products. Sugar is yeast's favourite food (ask anyone who makes wine or beer) and it makes sense not to feed it while you are trying to kill it with herbs and friendly bacteria.

Such methods are commonly extremely successful but may take three to six months (or more) to control the yeast overgrowth completely, although mouth and other local symptoms should show improvement within weeks.

It is all too common for people with Candida to have additional food sensitivities and allergies cause by the activity of the yeast in the intestines, which can have their delicate inner lining damaged by yeast so allowing absorption of undesirable substances that trigger the allergy reactions. For this reason extra care over diet is needed, avoiding anything that seems to provoke symptoms, especially if it is itself derived from yeasts or carries on it moulds.

Diet for Candida

Avoid all sugars and for the first few weeks avoid fruit as well. Avoid aged cheeses, dried fruits, any fermented products, including alcohol, and any food derived from or containing yeast.

Eat at least three ounces daily of fish, poultry or lean meat (free range only as many factory-farmed animals and fish contain antibiotic and steroid residues) unless you are vegetarian, in which case substitute grains and pulses and tofu (soy 'cheese') for this. Eat pulses (beans, lentils) and whole grains, especially rice, and abundantly of salad or lightly cooked vegetables.

Daily consumption of *live* cultured milk products (low fat if possible) such as yogurt or kefir is extremely helpful in Candida conditions – but avoid them if you are dairy sensitive. Make sure that such products contain live organisms and no sugar!

Supplements for Controlling Candida

Caprylic aid (coconut plant extract) capsules –
 two to four daily with meals.
Acidophilus and BifiDobacteria – a quarter
 teaspoonful of each (or one capsule) three

times daily away from meals in tepid water.
Garlic – three to six capsules daily with food.
Aloe vera juice – a teaspoon in a small tumbler
   of water several times a day. Additional help
   from other herbs requires expert advice.

Expect to feel slightly unwell for the first few days
of an anti-Candida diet as your body has to deal
with the dead yeast – you may feel flu-like
symptoms or nausea. Be patient and stick to the
programme for at least three months.

   If you have any tendency to Candida or other
infections in the mouth take extra care over
disinfecting toothbrushes and in any case start
using a new one at least once a month to prevent
reinfection, as brushes are a notorious have for
micro-organisms. An ideal toothpaste to use when
there is mouth Candida is one based on tea tree oil,
as this essential oil has strong antifungal properties.

   I have given a simple but far more thorough self-
help outline for dealing with Candida in my book
Candida Albicans – Could Yeast be Your Problem?
(Thorsons 1991).

OTHER BOWEL PARASITES

Another possible cause of body odour is the
presence in the intestines of parasites such as
worms and various protozoa. Self-help measures
for such conditions are sometimes very successful

but may be of only limited value in which case expert advice should be obtained. Signs of such problems include rectal itching (which can occur with Candida as well), loss of appetite and weight, anaemia, and a variety of colon disorders including diarrhoea or constipation or both (alternating).

Self-help measures include taking at least six garlic capsules a day in divided doses with food; and taking extract of grapefruit seeds (available from specialist health stores) and extract of pumpkin seeds, both of which encourage the expulsion of parasites. You should also follow the diet recommended for constipation (below).

CONSTIPATION

Sluggish bowel movements are one of the curses of civilised society and the cause of untold misery, with body odour being somewhere on the list of associated symptoms for many people. For the purposes of our consideration of the subject, constipation is a condition in which a person does not easily pass a bowel movement at least once a day.

Constipation simply means that the waste material passing through the bowel moves too slowly, leading to a build-up of gas, increased putrefaction of the material and the very real danger of possible absorption of extremely harmful toxic wastes – some of which may be expelled from the body via the skin, thereby causing body odour. Other side-effects of constipation include skin problems, a tendency to headaches, insomnia and bad breath. The risk of bowel cancer also increases dramatically with constipation, so the efforts to normalise this vital region's function should be seriously considered and scrupulously applied.

One of the main reasons for this increased risk of serious disease when there is chronic constipation is the effect it has on the billions of friendly bacteria living in our large and small intestines – an average of five pounds weight of these helpful bacteria live in each of us. When they are healthy, these friendly bacteria are active (among other useful jobs) in detoxifying the region, in return for which we house them and give them nourishment. However, if the 'food' they receive is excessively toxic or sugar laden, and fails to move along the digestive tract at a reasonable speed, the friendly bacteria can become inactive, damaged and relatively poor at doing the things they are supposed to do. And when this happens other nastier, less obliging organisms, such as yeasts and disease-causing bacteria, start colonising the regions in which the now weak and sluggish friendly bacteria live, leading to other problems – as we saw in our look at Candida. So in considering constipation we have to take account of the health of the friendly bacteria. Bifidobacteria inhabit the large intestines (including the colon) and Lactobacillus acidophilus lives in the small intestine (and mouth and vagina).

The primary reasons for constipation vary considerably from person to person, ranging from poor posture (causing crowding of the internal organs, which prevents them functioning normally) to lack of exercise, hormonal imbalances (pregnancy is a common time for constipation to appear), nervous system dysfunction (perhaps brought on by stress), the use of various medications (iron supplements, for example) and primarily – and most common of all – a diet that is out of balance and contains high levels of processed foods, such as white flour products, white rice and sugar, and only low levels of fibre.

Fibre is important because a diet rich in fibre produces a more rapid transit time of our food through our bodies – material stays for a shorter period inside us before elimination. However, there are problems associated with overuse of some forms of fibre, especially those derived from grains – their excessive use can produce a lot of gas, can reduce the absorption of nutrients from our food and can sometimes cause irritation of the bowel-wall. In general though, fibre improves bowel action through increasing bulk (water retention in the stool). This has the effect of stimulating the natural muscular action of the intestines (peristalsis) and a natural bowel movement should then take place without strain. Laxatives such as senna and various patent medications, on the other hand, irritate the bowel to open it, and this in the long run leads to the bowel becoming dependent on more and more irritation in order to get it to function at all.

Types of Fibre

The major sources of fibre in food are vegetables, grains (in the form of wheat bran) and pulses (beans).

The fibre in vegetables is excellent, and less irritating or likely to cause flatulence than bran. A medical study looking at the effects of different vegetable diets showed that the fibre from cabbage, carrots and apples produces similar effects to that gained by bran fibre but without the negative effects of possible irritation and gas. So a first step to fibre increase is simply to eat more fruit and vegetables.

A seed husk from the plant *plantago ovata* (psyllium) is widely used to increase the water retention of the stool, increasing its bulk and therefore helping to increase the speed of its elimination. Psyllium husks are available from health stores in their natural state – the forms of this seed sold by pharmacists usually contain sweetening or other chemical additives.

Naturally enough, if you are using something that increases the water retention of the stool, you also have to consume more liquid – surprisingly, many cases of constipation are caused simply through lack of adequate water intake. Not less than six pints of liquid should be consumed daily, in the form of water or juices. This can be reduced if a lot of fruit and raw vegetables are eaten, as the fluid content of plant foods is very high.

Many naturopaths believe that the best way of increasing fibre intake – apart from eating enough vegetables and fruit – is to use linseed (flaxseed). Linseed is a marvellous food in itself, containing important essential fatty acids, which we need for good health. It also has the property of absorbing liquid, so producing a bulky, gel-like, mass that passes through the intestine and stimulates peristalsis. It is the gel-like quality of the fibre of linseed that makes it so attractive when compared to the fibre of grains, which have a harsher quality.

Prescription for Bowel Health

1 Ensure that you eat a lot of vegetables, lightly cooked (stir-fried or steamed for preference), and fruit (paw paw, mango and avocado all contain excellent forms of fibre, as do apples, all the berries and pears). Avoid processed products as much as possible, especially white flour and white rice. Avoid sugar and make sure that you chew your food very well indeed. Avoid drinking with meals apart from a sip or two if essential.

2 Drink lots of spring water and juices – at least six pints daily on waking and between meals.

3 Take a dessertspoonful of linseed on its own, away from mealtimes, with a glass of water.

Put the seeds in your mouth, don't chew, just wash them down, and don't eat for at least a half an hour. If normal bowel movements have not started within a few days then increase the intake of linseed to twice a day (at separate times).

4 These measures will themselves help the friendly bacteria to function more normally. However, for the first six weeks of a programme to improve bowel health it is recommended that twice a day you also take, well away from mealtimes, the following friendly bacteria: a quarter teaspoonful of Bifidobacteria, together with a quarter teaspoonful of Lactobacillus acidophilus bacteria. At a separate time of day take Lactobacillus bulgaricus – a quarter teaspoonful with water.

5 For general bowel detoxification it is also suggested that you take with each meal one capsule of deodorised garlic oil.

6 As mentioned earlier, exercise and stress reduction are important factors in establishing regular bowel movements. Take a walk each day or perform some other regular, pleasant, non-competitive form of exercise. Avoid tension by practising some form of deep relaxation, ideally combined with breathing exercises. Perhaps join a yoga class or do this at home with the help of a book or video. See chapter 4 for more advice on this.

7 Never, ever, suppress the urge to go to the toilet. If you feel the urge, excuse yourself – whatever the situation – and go. Also avoid straining to pass a motion; if it does not come easily wait until it does. If you follow the advice above it won't be long before bowel movements are normal, and if body odour was directly connected with this it too should be much improved.

LOW BLOOD SUGAR

The main reason for including low blood sugar problems in this section is the fact that it leads to both excessive night sweats and 'cold sweating' whenever the sugar level drops.

There are a number of possible interacting causes of low blood sugar (hypoglycaemia). Symptoms can include headaches, extreme fatigue, depression, sleeplessness, phobic behaviour and panic attacks, inability to concentrate, cold sweats, allergic symptoms, dizziness, stomach pain, vision disorders, cold hands and feet, joint pains and many more. The condition will be accompanied by a craving for sweet food or stimulants such as tea, coffee, alcohol, tobacco or chocolate, which cause blood sugar to rise by stimulating the adrenal glands.

If any of these signs and symptoms are more noticeable when a meal has been missed then hypoglycaemia is likely – and if the symptoms are temporarily improved when sugar food or stimulants are used this is an almost certain sign. There are glucose tolerance tests which clearly prove hypoglycaemia, but the symptoms themselves are usually an accurate guide.

We store glucose (sugar) in the liver and muscles, and it is sent to the bloodstream rapidly when it is needed as a fuel. The body manufactures it from the food we eat, whether the foods are proteins or carbohydrates or fats. In order to keep levels of blood sugar just right, insulin is produced by the pancreas – and if your diet is balanced, and you are not using excessive stimulants, and your pancreas is working well, then your blood sugar levels remain balanced.

But if you are eating a great deal of sugar, sending blood sugar levels up rapidly and requiring insulin to control it, and if you are using stimulants excessively, which further keeps blood sugar levels shooting up (demanding more insulin), and if your stress levels are high, causing adrenalin to be released and more sugar to be shot into your bloodstream – then you can begin to sense that the controlling machinery is being strained. This series of swings between high and low blood sugar can occur when the sympathetic nervous system is out of balance with the parasympathetic – something we considered in chapter 4.

With these various influences we tend to get wild swings of sugar rising and falling, and with it mood-swings and feelings of exhaustion interspersed (when the sugar boost arrives) with a sense of being super-charged. Ultimately insulin control can collapse and diabetes (high blood sugar) can occur. In the meantime the range of symptoms listed above can develop, and one of these – cold sweats – interests us particularly since it can lead to body odour problems.

Help for Low Blood Sugar

Firstly, stimulants must be drastically reduced or stopped. This means nothing containing caffeine (including tea, coffee and chocolate), and no alcohol or tobacco use. A leading American practitioner, Michael Lesser MD, suggests that when hypoglycaemia is under control two cups of coffee daily can be allowed, as long as this is directly after meals.

For three months at least no sugar of any sort should be eaten in any form (jam, cakes, ice creams, etc.). Also to be avoided are all forms of refined (white) flour and white rice. Use fruit juices (apart from citrus and tomato) only sparingly, and then diluted 50:50 with water, as they can send blood sugar soaring.

Eat five or six snack meals daily instead of several large ones – and never miss breakfast.

Diet for Hypoglycaemia

BREAKFAST

Natural, low-fat yogurt and seeds, and nuts and grains or oatmeal porridge. Fresh fruit or wholewheat toast and low-fat cheese or an egg or fish (kipper). Drink coffee substitute or herbal tea.

TWO HOURS AFTER BREAKFAST

Fresh fruit, or natural yogurt, or skim milk drink, or nuts and seeds, or rice cakes.

LUNCH

Low-fat cheese, fish, poultry or vegetarian savoury and cooked or raw vegetables plus wholemeal bread or jacket potato.

TWO HOURS AFTER LUNCH

As mid-morning.

EARLY EVENING

If salad was eaten at midday eat a cooked meal now. If a cooked meal was eaten at midday have a salad with cottage cheese or yogurt.

BEFORE BED

As mid-morning and mid-afternoon.

Supplement with vitamin C (1 gram morning and evening) and vitamin B5 (pantothenic acid – 500 mg daily), zinc (30 mg daily) and chromium (1 mg daily). After three months a few liberties can be taken – but at the first sign of a return to the sugar-blues swings of mood go back to basics.

THE FISH-ODOUR SYNDROME

Some B.O. is extremely pungent, and has the smell of rotten fish. Milder versions of this particular problem also exist, and seem to relate to an inherited enzyme deficiency which is aggravated by disturbed bowel flora and particular foods.

Studies in London have shown that diet is a specific irritant in this usually inherited condition, which seems to affect only a small percentage of people with B.O. Only 11 out of 156 people who wrote to the researchers about their body odour problems had the syndrome. (*British Medical Journal*, 11 September 1993, pp.655-657.)

When we eat particular foods rich in certain biochemical compounds such as the amino acid carnitine, any residues that remain in the intestines to be worked on by the natural flora (friendly bacteria) require particular enzymes to break them down to an odourless state for the body to excrete in the urine. If the enzymes are deficient, or if the friendly bacteria manufacture too much of these materials (specifically carnitine and choline), the characteristic rotten-fish odour is produced. Other factors that make this problem worse are stress, anxiety and menstruation – some women are more affected if they are taking the contraceptive pill at the time.

The guidelines given in chapter 6 regarding detoxification, as well as the advice given about diet and Candida on pages 31–38, should be looked at carefully in order to help normalise intestinal flora and remove toxic debris from the system. A balanced diet as outlined in chapter 8 is also called for, but particular foods should be avoided by people with 'fish-odour syndrome'.

The foods that lead to excessive presence of carnitine are those rich in the amino acid lysine, and these include:

Meat
Potatoes
Milk
Brewer's yeast
Fish
Chicken
Beans
Eggs

The foods that lead to excessive levels of choline are those rich in lecithin, and these include:

Eggs
Soya products
Corn
Wheatgerm

These foods are those which supply the raw

material for fish-odour syndrome and they should be kept to only modest levels in the diet, with greater emphasis on eating vegetables, grains such as rice, and fruit. This does not mean that the foods listed above should never be eaten, only that they should be eaten in smaller quantities than in the past.

Anyone with fish-odour syndrome should also supplement regularly with Lactobacillus acidophilus and Bifidobacteria as outlined on page 37. The need for keeping stress levels low is also important for people with this problem – see pages 20–30. True fish-odour syndrome is probably the worst sort of B.O., but it affects a relatively small number of people. Nevertheless, anyone with persistent B.O. should consider a diet low in lecithin and lysine for a month or so to assess the affects on their condition.

All of these conditions – Candida, bowel parasites, constipation, hypoglycaemia and fish-odour syndrome – can lead to body odour. It is quite possible to suffer from several of these problems at the same time and if this is the case professional advice should be sought. Additionally, various liver conditions and diabetes can lead to body odour, and these conditions – while benefiting from the general advice in this book – also require expert attention.

If none of these conditions apply to you and your current health status, and if you have body odour problems, then read the next chapter on detoxification.

CHAPTER SIX

How to Detoxify Using Nutrition and Water Therapy

Our bodies constantly detoxify themselves – of the by-products of life produced all the time by our cells, as well as of the toxic accumulations that we acquire from our food and water, the air we breathe, and from medications and drugs. The neutralisation of toxins is taken care of by our immune system, by 'friendly bacteria' living in our bowels and by our liver and kidneys, and the wastes produced in the detoxification process leave the body via the urine, the faeces, the air we breathe out and in our perspiration.

The number of chemicals that can be found in each and every one of us, many of which should not be present even in minute traces, is profoundly worrying and hazardous to our health. It is now known that *everyone* on the planet has deposits in their tissues of DDT, lead, cadmium and dioxin. The chances are therefore that a wide range of petro-chemical by-products, as well as heavy metals, food additives, colourings, flavourings, preservatives, insecticides and pesticides are all present in most of us to some extent.

We have become filters and traps for pollutants that exist in ever greater amounts all around us. These pollutants have a definite effect on our overall health, as well as imposing increasing demands on our organs of elimination – one of which is the function of perspiring. Healthy organs of elimination combined with a sound immune system can work wonders even with this sort of toxic load, but in time our bodies can become less efficient and we should consider giving a helping hand to the detoxification process.

The toxic build-up in our bodies is greater when we are stressed. For example, if muscles are held tensely they create and retain acid wastes. These can be flushed away by exercise and fresh oxygenated blood and they can also be excreted through the skin as sweat, *or* they can be retained in the tissues due to sluggish circulation and poor oxygenation caused by inadequate exercise and breathing. If toxins are retained they can become irritants and interfere with normal function. Reducing tension and adding in exercise and deep breathing along with methods for increasing elimination through the skin (such as the water therapy methods described later in this chapter) will all therefore reduce this part of your toxic burden.

All our organs of detoxification need to be well nourished in order to work efficiently – well supplied with fresh oxygenated blood carrying adequate nutrient supplies and served by a nervous system that is working correctly. As we get older, and when we are exposed to a greater degree of toxicity and stress from many sources, so our ability to self-cleanse – to detoxify – becomes less efficient, as do our various supporting functions such as circulation and elimination. We all carry a greater or lesser load of this undesirable debris stored in our tissues (mainly in our fat stores below the skin). And this is added to daily by exposure to new toxic materials in food, water and the air we breathe, not to forget any extra toxicity we create or acquire through infection or from certain forms of medication.

No-one has a clear idea of just what damage all this is doing to us, especially when you consider the combination of these toxic materials interacting as they do with the very real individual biochemical differences we are each born with and the huge differences that exist between people in terms of their levels of nutritional, structural and emotional excellence or deficiency. Some of us handle the toxic load better than others, but in the end all of us are negatively affected, sometimes with profound consequences to the levels of health we enjoy or the sort and intensity of the illnesses we suffer. And in some of us the elimination through the skin of toxic wastes adds to the likelihood of body odour.

The best way of handling this sort of situation is to decrease the toxic burden, to encourage increased elimination, and to find ways of reducing future build-up of toxic accumulation.

HELPING YOURSELF

The need for each of us to tackle these toxic burdens before they actually produce health problems has never been greater. The good news is that there is an enormous amount each of us can do to help ourselves. Not only can we ensure a balanced diet, but we can make sure we get enough of the right sort of exercise – and we can take care of the vital area which controls everything else – our emotional well-being and ability to cope with stress. We can also work at regularly cleansing the system ourselves, with hydrotherapy as a key part of this process.

Many scientists believe that the future of health care will have at its very core an absolute requirement for safe and effective detoxification procedures, and hopefully these can be started before our immune system and vital organs have started to decline in efficiency.

Before looking at the ways in which various safe and easy-to-apply water treatments can assist in detoxification we should consider other ways of ridding ourselves of impurities. If body odour is a feature of your life then the chances are that your body's elimination and detoxification functions are operating at less than their optimum. Fortunately a number of methods for safe home use exist which can encourage elimination of impurities. These include repetitive short fasting periods which allow the liver in particular to recover from toxic stress. A number of variations on the theme of fasting are explained and outlined in this chapter.

GENTLE DETOXIFICATION PROGRAMMES

If you are robust and vital a more vigorous detoxification program will be needed than if you are unwell and somewhat fragile in your health. The following detox programme is safe for almost everyone – but do check with your health adviser first.

NOTE

If you are a recovering drug user or alcoholic or have an eating disorder or are a diabetic then do not *apply these methods without asking professional advice first. If you have Candida or bowel problems or are hypoglycaemic then use self-help or professional guidance to help normalise these conditions before starting on the detoxification methods listed below.*

NUTRITIONAL DETOXIFICATION

Priority number one in detoxification is dietary. Over almost *every* weekend for a few months, and thereafter once a month at least, choose between a short water-only fast and a full weekend monodiet.

Short Water-Only Fast

This is conducted over a weekend, starting Friday evening and ending Saturday evening or Sunday morning, or just all day Saturday, so that work schedules are not interfered with. Make sure that you drink not less than four and not more than eight pints of water during the day.

After fasting for 24 to 36 hours break the fast with stewed pears or apples (no sweetening), or with a light vegetable soup, or with plain, low-fat unsweetened yogurt. On the Sunday have a raw food day, with fruit or salad only, well chewed. Or, if you have a sensitive digestion, have lightly cooked vegetables (steamed or stir fried), a baked potato and stewed fruit (no sugar) plus yogurt. Drink as much water as you like.

A Full Weekend Monodiet

Start this on Friday night and go through to Sunday evening. The idea is that you eat just one food throughout the weekend. You can have up to three pounds daily of any single fruit, such as grapes, apples, pears (best choice if you have a history of allergy) or papaya (ideal if you have digestive problems). Alternatively, have brown rice or buckwheat or millet or potatoes (skin and all), boiled and eaten whenever desired. You can eat up to a pound dry weight of any of the grains once they have been cooked, made palatable by the addition of a little lemon juice and olive oil, or three pounds of potatoes daily. If you choose fruit only then it can be raw or lightly stewed without sweetening.

Whichever type of weekend detox you choose make sure you rest and keep warm and have no engagements or dates. This is a time to allow all available energy to focus on the repairing and cleansing processes of detoxification.

Midweek Programme

In between these weekend detoxification intensives you can follow a milder midweek programme of detoxification.

BREAKFAST

Fresh fruit (raw or lightly cooked – no sweetening) and live yogurt, *or* home-made muesli (seeds and nuts and grains) and live yogurt, *or* cooked grains and yogurt (buckwheat, millet, linseed, barley, rice, etc.). Drink herbal tea (linden blossom, chamomile, mint, sage, lemon verbena) or lemon and hot water.

LUNCH AND SUPPER

One of these should be a raw salad with jacket potato or brown rice and either bean curd (tofu) or low-fat cheese or nuts and seeds. Or, if raw food is a problem, have a stir-fried vegetable and tofu meal or steamed vegetables eaten with potato or rice, together with low-fat cheese or nuts and seeds.

The other main meal should be a choice between fish, chicken, game or a vegetarian savoury (a pulse and grain combination) and vegetables lightly steamed, baked or stir fried.

DESSERTS

Lightly stewed fruit – add apple or lemon juice (not sugar) or live natural yogurt.

Season food with garlic and herbs, avoiding salt as much as possible. Eat slowly, chew well, don't drink with meals and consume at least two pints of liquid daily between meals. Take one high-potency multimineral/multivitamin capsule daily and three garlic capsules. Also take daily an acidophilus supplement for bowel detox support.

What to Expect During Detoxification

For the first few weekends of short-term fasting or monodiet you could develop a headache and furred tongue, and during the weekend body odour may be even stronger than usual – this is normal and acceptable. All these side effects of detoxification – which tell you that the process is working – will slowly get less obvious as detoxification progresses weekend by weekend. *Take nothing to stop the headache, just rest as much as you can.*

As the weeks pass your skin should become clearer (it may get a bit spotty for a while), your eyes clearer, your brain sharper, your digestion more efficient, your energy levels should rise and you should regain a feeling of youthful clarity you had forgotten and body odour problems should get less and less.

When your tongue no longer becomes furred with the weekend detox and headaches no longer appear you can begin to spread these intensive detox weekends apart – three a month and then two a month and then maintenance of once a month. When you notice a definite change, and less reaction to the weekend fasts, the in-between, milder detoxification pattern can also be relaxed a bit with the inclusion of a few 'naughty but nice' tasty toxins from time to time, allowing your social life to be a bit more relaxed. By this time your internal detox system should be able to cope with such indiscretions!

Additional Detoxification Support

While you are on this safe detoxification programme a variety of other methods to assist detoxification can be added into your self-help programme. These include

- Epsom salt baths or wet sheet packs (see pages 69–73 for details) – once weekly
- Skin brushing to assist skin elimination (see page 63) – daily
- Stretching and relaxation exercises – daily
- Brisk aerobic exercise (walking, jogging, skipping, rebounding, dancing, work-out) – every day except during the fasting period and only if appropriate to your health
- Essential aromatherapy oils in your baths as described on pages 74–78
- Breathing relaxation and meditation methods (see pages 23–27) – every day at least once for 10-15 minutes, twice would be better

DETOXIFICATION THROUGH WATER THERAPY

You and Your Skin

Your skin is not just the envelope that surrounds you, it is a powerful organ. Your skin is a 'second lung' through which your body eliminates a great deal of waste material – when it is healthy, that is. Your circulatory system carries metabolic wastes (produced normally as by-products of your normal body functions) to the skin along tiny capillaries where they pass out of you through the pores. The outer surface of the skin itself is made up of 'dead' cells which you shed all the time, but when these dead skin cells become covered with micro-scopically small dirt particles and oils (which you produce yourself) the easy elimination processes of the body through the pores of the skin can be blocked or slowed, leading to blemishes, pimples and blackheads and also to reduced ease of sweat-ing – which is vital for adequate detoxification.

Benefits of Detoxifying

A number of benefits to your general health can derive from techniques to ensure that your skin is working efficiently, because your level of toxicity drops, putting less strain on other organs of elimination such as the liver, kidneys, bowels and lungs. In fact minor problems such as chronic catarrh can improve or vanish when the skin becomes more efficient with open channels instead of blocked ones. This is because when the skin does its job properly there is less need for other means of removal of toxins, such as excretion through the mucous membranes. And any tendency to unpleasant body odour will also reduce dramatic-ally with the self-treatments described below.

SKIN CARE AND TREATMENTS IN YOUR HOME

To get your skin functioning efficiently you need to work on its surface as well as stimulating circulation to and through it. Methods that focus largely on skin include

- Skin brushing (dry method and wet method)
- Salt glow
- Peat bath
- Epsom salts bath
- Wet sheet pack

To stimulate overall circulation to your skin as well as improving its function, the following whole-body 'systemic' methods are suggested

- Sauna (ideally followed by a cold dip)
- Aromatherapy baths (using specific oils as described on pages 74–78)

Skin Brushing

DRY METHOD

This is best done 'dry' before you wash, shower or bathe, and it need take only a few minutes (five at most). Once you decide to start using skin brushing to improve your skin and health you should also make up your mind that it will become a daily routine – and because it makes you feel so good (never mind looking good) very soon you will feel as lost without it as you would if you forgot to brush your teeth!

Buy a bath-mit or a loofah or a natural bristle body-brush. Make sure the room is warm and there are no draughts, because you need to have no clothes on to do this job effectively. It can be done standing but sitting on a stool allows you to deal with the backs of your legs and other 'difficult' parts more efficiently, without having to perform contortions.

You should start brushing gently and at first expect what is called a 'red reaction', which shows that your circulation is responding to the stimulation you are giving it. The action of brushing needs to be circular, 'creeping' and firm but not irritating. The circular motion helps you avoid rubbing over one area too much (at first once or twice over any part of the skin is adequate) and the 'creeping' has the same effect. This simply means that you gradually move from where you are circling to the next area, not by lifting the brush but by altering the direction as you make the circular motion, and so slide gently towards the next part of the skin that is due to receive attention.

Pay particular attention to the skin on the backs of your legs and arms as well as to your back, abdomen and chest, where you may be more sensitive and tender. Women should avoid breast tissue and be very gentle on the inner thighs.

Again it is emphasised that you should start slowly and gently. After a week or so of skin brushing the skin that was tender will be less so and you can slowly increase the pressure and vigour of your brushing.

If there are bits of your back you cannot reach use

a dry towel to briskly friction this area – it will not be as effective as a brush or loofah, but it will be better than no friction at all.

WET METHOD

For skin brushing using the alternative wet method, choose from the same forms of brush (a mit or loofah or natural bristle skin brush). First shower or bathe, and before drying perform the process as described for dry brushing but moisten the brush as well. Shower afterwards to get rid of any surface skin that has been loosened by the process, ideally finishing with water that is around body temperature or cooler.

Salt Glow

The salt glow is a skin friction using wet coarse (sea) salt or Epsom salts. It is particularly beneficial if you have difficulty sweating or have poor circulation to your hands and/or feet and it is also useful if you are prone to rheumatic aches and pains.

If you have a B.O. problem it can derive from a general deficiency in sweating, with most of it taking place in just a few areas such as the underarms. By using the salt glow (and skin brushing as above) you will encourage the rest of the body's surface to behave more normally.

The salt glow is best done to you, and for self-treatment it is necessary to accept that bits of your body are not going to be reached – just imagine trying to effectively friction *all* of your back yourself! Unlike the skin brushing method, which is suggested as a daily routine, the salt glow is a now-and-then thing – perhaps once a week at most if you have difficulty sweating and once a month or so for general detoxification purposes.

MATERIALS
You will need a bowl and at least a half pound of coarse salt or Epsom salts.

METHOD
Sit on a stool in the bath or shower and add water to the salt in the bowl to moisten it – just enough to make the salt grains stick together. Take a small amount of wet salt into each hand (a tablespoonful approximately) and starting with one foot work the salt into the skin as you come up the leg using up and down and circular motions. Try to friction firmly, even vigorously, on skin that is usually exposed, such as the legs, as you apply the damp salt so that all the skin gets some rubbing and some salt. Work up each leg and then do each arm. Next work the salt into the skin around your back without straining yourself (if your partner is handy they could usefully do all the frictioning for you – or at least the back). Then apply the salt, rubbing firmly but not irritatingly, to the abdomen and

chest and up to the neck (avoid breast tissues).

After the salt rub you need to shower *thoroughly*, ideally using a hand shower and warm water to cleanse the surface of the skin. As you are doing this and the water is playing on a given area, use your free hand to rub the salt and water off the skin, giving the area a bit more friction as you do so. Dry with a vigorous towelling down and go to bed – make sure it and the room are warm.

You should sleep very well and may perspire heavily after the first few times you use the salt glow. Have water by the bed in case you get thirsty. As your skin becomes more efficient so will this heavy perspiration lessen as time passes. This is a wonderful skin tonic and detoxification method.

Peat Bath

When you use peat in a bath you are adding the combined concentrated material of hundreds and thousands of years of compression of the organic materials from decaying mosses, leaves and roots. The resulting 'soup' contains rich supplies of silica, sulphur, iron, resins and many minerals and harmless acids.

Many of these ingredients help to neutralise harmful toxins on and under the skin and, since many of the micro-elements in peat can be absorbed through the skin, these can also influence your general health, with particular benefits to skin and rheumatic problems. Medical research has also shown that peat baths can help blood pressure problems, circulatory difficulties and in restoring balance when there are sugar disturbances. Use of a peat bath now and then as well as the regular use of skin brushing is an excellent way of improving skin function.

MATERIALS
You need liquid peat or Austrian moor material.

METHOD
The very best way of using this black organic material is to apply it as a paste to the body surface as a whole, and while this done effectively at health spas it is not a practical proposition in the home. By using liquid peat or moor you can enjoy the health benefits at home. All you need do is pour the liquid (amounts will be indicated on the container) into a hot bath and soak for between 20 and 30 minutes. Shower well afterwards and retire to a warm bed.

Just as in the case of the salt glow you might expect to perspire more than usual that might and sleep very well indeed. Have water by your bed to make up the liquid lost through sweating, and be prepared to change your sheets next morning. If you are rheumatic and have an acidic tendency then a peat bath every week would be a good idea.

Epsom Salts Bath

There are few more effective ways of stimulating skin function than an Epsom salts bath. It dramatically increases elimination through the skin and, as in the case of the peat bath, is ideal if there is any tendency towards acidity, rheumatic problems or if there is a need to detoxify – as there certainly is in most people with body odour problems.

NOTE

Anyone with a serious cardiac condition or diabetes, or a skin condition that is 'open' or weeping, should not use this method. If you are pregnant or have high blood pressure, get clearance from your medical practitioner first.

MATERIALS

You need Epsom salts, sea salt, iodine and a bath.

METHOD

Into a hot (comfortably hot – not scalding) bath place one pound of commercial Epsom salts (from any good pharmacy) plus a quarter to a half pound of sea salt and a dessertspoonful of iodine (get the clear variety to avoid staining the bath). This combination of salt and iodine approximates the constituents of the sea. Stay in the bath (you just lie there as it is quite impossible to wash in the salt mixture) for not less than 10 minutes and not more than 20. Top up with hot water if you stay in beyond 10 minutes to keep the water feeling hot. When you get out do not shower – just towel yourself dry and get into a pre-warmed bed.

Once again, as with the peat bath and the salt glow, you should expect to sweat heavily – and to sleep even more heavily. Have water by the bed as you may need to top up the lost liquid. In the morning take a shower and apply a moisturiser to the skin as a whole.

It is not recommended that you take an Epsom salts bath more than once a week, and once a month is probably the ideal for general detoxification purposes and stimulation of skin function.

Wet Sheet Pack

The way a wet sheet pack works depends on how you use it. The full sheet pack passes through four distinct stages of activity, each of which has a different effect on the person receiving it. Described simply these four states are:

1 An initial cooling stage, useful for feelings of general weakness or if there is a fever. This stage lasts no more than five minutes.
2 A neutral stage, when the pack is the same

temperature as the body, which helps calm agitation, anxiety and nervousness. This stage may last for half an hour or more depending upon how quickly your body heat warms the material containing the water.

3 A hot stage, which helps in a number of health conditions but which is more useful for pain problems such as sinus congestion, bowel discomfort (especially if constipated) or conditions such as colitis.

4 A stage when sweating becomes profuse, which is used for detoxification – anything from general detoxification to eliminating the residue of drugs (including tobacco), alcohol or during some infections to hasten the fever process (under supervision only).

NOTE

Avoid stages three and four if you are very anaemic or very weak or debilitated. Being wrapped, mummy-like, can be claustrophobic so there should always be someone handy to help with removal of the pack in case this happens or if you feel unwell. Do not use a wet sheet pack if you have a skin condition that is made worse by water. Anyone with diabetes should take advice before using a wet sheet pack.

MATERIALS

You need two cotton sheets, two wool blankets, towels, a pillow, a hot water bottle and a hand towel.

METHOD

This treatment is impossible to do for yourself so someone has to help with the application.

Place a blanket on the bed, open fully. Have a warm shower and on emerging from this have someone ready to wrap you in a cold, wet sheet which should have been wrung out in water at between 60 and 70°F (15–21°C). Working swiftly, this should be wrapped from under your armpits so that it fits snugly to your body right down to the ankles, and should be immediately covered by a second sheet (dry) before you lie down onto the blanket, which should be wrapped around you from neck to feet with no sheet being allowed to be visible (thus avoiding access to air which would keep it cool). The second blanket should be placed over the first one and tucked around you snugly.

Use towels and/or a neck pillow to insulate areas such as the neck where the blanket may not be enclosing the pack efficiently. Place a hot water bottle near the feet. Speed of operation is essential as chilling will occur if the work is done slowly.

When the third or fourth stages are reached (it feels hot and/or you start to sweat), a cold compress to the forehead is a good idea, as would be the offer of sips of water if you feel thirsty (sweating can be profuse in stage four so water replenishment is needed).

The pack can be discontinued at or after any of the four stages as appropriate. For full benefit it should run its course, which takes up to three hours or more depending upon your vitality (how quickly you heat the sheet). If at any time after the first few minutes the pack is uncomfortably cold it should be stopped and a brisk friction applied to the whole body surface using a mitten or dry towel to stimulate circulation. The failure of the sheet to warm up would indicate either that the sheet was too wet or the water too cold, or that the insulation was inadequately applied.

Sauna Bathing for Overall Health

Another method that encourages more normal skin function is the Scandinavian concept of dry heat followed by a cold plunge or shower. Unless you have the resources at home, you will have to visit a health club or sauna bath.

Why would you want to increase sweating when B.O. is the result of sweating anyway? As we have seen there are a number of excellent ways in which the skin can be encouraged to function more efficiently in its elimination tasks, and a sauna bath is designed to achieve just this end. By periodically cleansing the pores and making the sweat glands work overtime, the chance of clearing waste products from the body increases. A sauna also has profound relaxing effects.

Ideally a short-term exposure to the intense dry heat of the sauna followed by a cold shower or plunge several times a month is called for – more if you like it and can afford it. At first don't stay in the sauna for more than 10 minutes, on the lower benches where heat is slightly less intense. After this have a shower or plunge and rest for 20 minutes or so. The next time you go stay a little longer (not more than 15 minutes) and perhaps venture onto the higher benches. Again finish with a tepid then cool or cold shower and dip and a rest.

If you wish to treat yourself to an aromatherapy massage after this you will feel fantastic.

NOTE

Do *not* have a sauna bath if you are pregnant or have a serious heart condition or high blood pressure without first obtaining medical clearance.

Aromatherapy Baths

The selection of oils described below have proven herbal properties. None are meant to be consumed. When added to a bath the oils are used neat in the running water, which disperses and mixes them. Store essential oils, individually or in combinations, in clean glass containers (dark if possible) away from light, tightly capped. The various indications given for each oil, and combinations of oils, can help you select the one(s) most useful for your present state of health.

BASIL

Its properties include it being an antiseptic as well as an antidepressant and a tonic for the digestion. On its own it can be used to treat weakness, fatigue (including mental tiredness and fogginess), headaches, nausea, feelings of tension or faintness and depression. Use it with neroli (10 drops of each in a bath) for relaxing you.

CHAMOMILE

Its properties include it being a soothing agent, sleep enhancer, digestive and general tonic, pain reliever and an antibacterial agent. It can be used on its own to treat sleep and digestive disturbances, skin conditions, neuralgia, and inflammation. It soothes tired and irritated eyes when used as a compress or eyewash. Combine it with sage for menopausal problems (10 drops of each in a bath),

CYPRESS

This is an astringent, antispasmodic, tonic and is useful as a deodorant. It can be used alone to treat rheumatic and muscular conditions, coughs, flu and nervous tension. Combined with lemon oil, a drop of the mixture is applied (neat) to acne spots and skin discolouration. Combine it with lavender (20 drops of each in warm water) for menopausal problems or for general nervous system treatment.

LAVENDER

This is an antispasmodic, antiseptic and general restorative. It acts as an insect repellant. It is used alone to treat nervous problems, skin lesions such as burns and wounds, and acne. It makes a useful douche. Use it alone for headaches (20 drops or oil in a bath). Use it with chamomile (20 drops of each in a tepid bath) for sunburn, with cypress (as above) for menopausal or 'nervous system' problems and with vetiver for anxiety.

NEROLI

This is an antidepressant, antiseptic, digestive aid as well as being said to be both a sedative and aphrodisiac. It is used alone (20 drops in a bath) to treat depression, insomnia and nervous tension, digestive upsets and lack of sexual interest. It is a skin enhancing agent. Use it together with basil (10 drops of each in a bath) in cases of anxiety, tension or depression.

ROSE

Its properties include it being antibacterial, antidepressant, aphrodisiac, astringent, sedative and a tonic for the heart and liver. It has specific influences on the female reproductive organs, especially the uterus. Alone (20 drops in a bath) it is used to treat depression, poor sex drive, headache, nausea and insomnia, as well as being useful for douching and as a skin tonic.

SAGE

This is a tonic, antiseptic and diuretic, which influences the female reproductive system and blood pressure. Alone (20 drops in a bath) it is used to treat nervousness, fatigue, chest complaints, menopausal problems, low blood pressure and is useful as a douche. Use it together with chamomile in menopausal problems.

SANDALWOOD

This is an antiseptic, aphrodisiac and tonic. It is used alone (20 drops in a bath) to treat bronchitis, urinary infections impotence and fatigue.

VETIVER

This is a calming agent and is used alone (20 drops in a bath) to treat anxiety and nervous conditions.

Use it with lavender for anxiety and tension (10 drops of each in a bath).

If you combine regular (daily) skin brushing and a periodic (weekly, or at least twice a month) salt glow or Epsom salt baths and/or moor baths, with a sauna now and then and a luxurious aroma-therapy bath whenever you want one the important process of skin normalisation and body detoxification will be greatly helped. You will find most of these methods extremely relaxing and pleasant as well. These methods are meant to be used together with nutritional detoxification – not instead of it.

Detoxification is vital for general health enhancement as well as for dealing with many of the underlying causes of body odour and the recommendation is that *at least three months* be given over to using the methods outlined in this chapter.

By using the fasting detox methods you are providing the body with an opportunity to correct a great many problems about which you may be completely unaware. Fasting is a period of what is called 'physiological rest' during which our internal self-healing mechanisms speed up their normal activities. You will therefore find that skin problems improve, circulation improves, digestive problems ease or vanish, your eyes are able to function more efficiently, your sense of smell is keener, you have more energy, and so on through the various body systems and functions.

At the end of three months of applying the methods suggested in this chapter most people should – depending on the level of toxicity at the outset – be able to reduce their detox weekends to a once a month maintenance level.

CHAPTER SEVEN

Why You May Need to Take Supplements

Because supplements are recommended in this book in order to help specific conditions associated with body odour, we have to ask a very vexed question. *Why should some people have different nutritional requirements from others?*

The recommended daily allowance (RDA) of any particular vitamin or mineral is set by a panel of scientific advisers to governments and is thought by them to meet the essential needs of all 'healthy people'. Even if it is accepted that this RDA level is accurate for healthy people – and this is strongly contested by many nutritionists as being inadequately low in most cases – there are many people who do not fit into the category of 'essentially healthy'. Are you one of them? You might well require additional nutritional support, beyond what you are supposed to be getting from your food, in order to maintain health if certain conditions apply to you. You will probably need to take supplements if you:

- have a very large or very small body size
- live in a hot climate or work in a hot environment
- are under stress at work
- have wounds, burns or other injuries
- are taking prescribed medication
- have digestive problems
- are pregnant or a nursing mother
- have an unusual or unique metabolism
- have a chronic illness
- are involved in heavy regular exercise (training, aerobics, etc.)
- regularly consume alcohol *or* smoke
- regularly consume coffee
- are involved in regular dieting or slimming
- are past retirement age
- are going through puberty
- use oral contraceptives
- have infections
- have too little or no exercise
- are exposed to radiation (even sun-bathing)
- consume polluted water (i.e. most tap-water)
- are exposed to polluted air or pesticides
- are under emotional stress

Even if you do not fit into one of these categories there is another unhappy fact to absorb: that detailed surveys of almost all population groups, including young children, school children, teenagers, young adults, middle-aged individuals in all socio-economic groups and the elderly, regularly show that between 80 and 90 per cent *fail to receive in their daily diet all the RDA of essential nutrients.* And this comes on top of the established fact that before we even start to consider the individual circumstances listed above, we all begin with different nutritional requirements because of genetic programming. This is known medically as 'biochemical individuality' and it means that in the case of each of the nearly 50 different nutrients (vitamins etc.) that we need to survive in good health there will be variations in need from person to person – by up to 700 per cent in many instances.

Nutritionists and naturopaths find that in most cases of ill health some dietary adjustment, and often supplementation, is needed to help recovery. In an ideal world we should get all our nutrients from our food, but we don't – or at least most of us don't – and so supplementation becomes a useful safety net, a health insurance strategy, for health maintenance and disease prevention. It becomes a necessity when we are out of balance sufficiently to be manifesting symptoms of ill health in a chronic way – and body odour is evidence of such an imbalance.

CHAPTER EIGHT

General Nutrition and Nutritional Supplementation

If you have no particular health problems such as Candida, constipation or low blood sugar, and yet you have B.O., a general balanced diet should be adopted after you have followed the detoxification programme until your tongue is no longer furred and your detox reaction (headache etc.) is much less obvious than previously.

GENERAL GUIDELINES FOR OPTIMUM NUTRITION

The following guidelines are useful for everyone:

- Eat whole food – as 'dense' (requiring chewing because it is as close to unprocessed as possible) as is manageable with as few additives as possible.
- Eat organic and fresh vegetables, fruits and proteins (fish and meat) whenever available.
- Reduce or eliminate simple sugars and replace with

- complex carbohydrates (vegetables, whole grains, beans, etc.) which are rich in nutrients such as zinc.
- Reduce polyunsaturated and saturated fats and oils.
- Use mono-unsaturated oils instead (olive oil).
- Eat little and often throughout the day to optimise absorption of nutrients from food (see pages 47–48).
- Try to keep a balance of food intake which ensures 65 per cent is complex carbohydrates (vegetables, fruits, pulses, grains), 15 per cent is protein (fish, yogurt, eggs, meat) and 20 per cent is fat.
- Make sure vegetables are thoroughly clean and free of parasites and bacteria by steaming lightly and/or washing very thoroughly before eating.
- Eat a wide variety of foods.
- Avoid altogether chocolate, caffeine and alcohol.

A Sample Day's Diet

BREAKFAST

Choose *two or three* selections from

Mixed seeds (sunflower, pumpkin, sesame, linseed) and grains (wheat, oat, millet, rice flakes). The seeds can be eaten whole or milled in a coffee grinder. The grains and seeds can be lightly oven-roasted or soaked overnight in a little water to soften them, and eaten with live low-fat yogurt and fresh fruit or on their own.

Oat (or millet) porridge plus fresh almonds or walnuts.

Vegetable or fish soup with whole rice or noodles
Live low-fat yogurt or kefir
Sourdough rye or wheat bread or toast with
  olive oil or cottage cheese (low fat) or egg.
Enzyme-rich fruit such as papaya.
Tofu (bean curd) stir fried with vegetables
Two or three eggs weekly (boiled, poached or
  scrambled).
Drink herbal teas or spring water.

MID-MORNING AND MID-AFTERNOON SNACKS

Rich cakes or any of the items listed under
'breakfast'.

LUNCH AND EVENING MEAL

Unless a vegetarian diet has been chosen one, at
least, of these meals should contain an animal
protein such as fish, free-range poultry (no skin) or
game (to avoid the antibiotics and steroids given to
most farm-reared animals). If fish is chosen then a
cold-water type such as herring, salmon, sardine,
haddock, sole or cod should be eaten. Cook by
boiling, steaming, grilling, casseroling, stir-frying,
poaching or use in a soup. Avoid frying or roasting
as this alters nature of any fat content.

  Ideally protein should be eaten with green
vegetables and/or seaweed (from Oriental or health
stores) which are lightly cooked in one of the ways
mentioned.

Seasoning should be by use of herbs, garlic and spices with as little salt as possible, or with Oriental seasoning such as miso. If any oil is employed in cooking it should be virgin olive oil which can also be used as a dressing.

The other main meal should be similar or could be based on a combination of pulses (chickpeas, mung beans, lentils, kidney beans or any other sort of bean) and grains (millet, brown rice, quinoa, amaranth, buckwheat, etc., whole or as pasta or noodles). A soup, stew, roast or other combination of these ingredients provides a first-class protein source. Low-fat cheese (cottage, for example) or tofu can also be eaten at this time.

A variety of starchy vegetables (lightly cooked) such as carrot, beet, squash or potato, as well as green vegetables, are also highly desirable. There is abundant evidence of the health-enhancing value of brassica (cabbage, kale, broccoli). If your digestion is good include raw salads as well.

Desserts should be low-fat live yogurt or enzyme-rich fruit such as papaya, apple or pear.

THE MODIFIED MAYR CURE

This is a healthy eating plan that will improve vitality and general health. Periodically, say once a year, it is an excellent idea to introduce a one, two or three-week 'Mayr Cure' diet. This Austrian concept encourages a more efficient digestion by retraining you into sound eating habits. It is an excellent way of losing weight, but more importantly it improves the way we handle food, ensuring that we absorb more from the food we eat and at the same time placing less strain on our digestive functions.

Re-education of the digestive system seems in many instances to be possible if you follow a diet that demands a greater degree of chewing than is normal. You are asked systematically to chew each mouthful of food between 40 and 50 times, so that whatever is being eaten becomes a paste. The diet may sound unattractive, but it is effective.

Breakfast should comprise a three-day-old (stale) dry roll or one that has been 'dried' in a warm oven. Take only small bites of this, *with no fluid at all*. Chew each mouthful as per the guidelines above. This stimulates the 'satiety' centre in your brain (which tells you when you have had enough to eat) as well as mixing enzymes with the food. When each mouthful has become a paste, place one teaspoonful of plain low-fat live yogurt in your mouth with this paste and chew a few more times, and then swallow.

In this way you will eat approximately a quarter of a tub of live yogurt and a stale roll for breakfast. Drink nothing and eat nothing else.

Not less than half an hour after the roll and yogurt, drink a herbal tea such as fennel, sage, lemon verbena, linden blossom, chamomile or peppermint.

For lunch have a variety of lightly cooked vegetables (steamed or stir-fried) together with fish or lean meat, but before eating this start the meal with another dry roll.

In the evening have a dry roll, yogurt and cooked vegetables. Start the meal with the dry roll and yogurt, and then have the vegetables. Drink a herbal tea at least half an hour later.

During the day sip pure water only apart from the herbal teas, and during the two weeks of the modified Mayr Cure eat no fruit, no raw vegetables, no fatty food, no alcohol or coffee and absolutely no sugar. The amount of time spent chewing is what determines how successful the programme will be.

SUPPLEMENTATION

A number of nutrients have been found to be extremely effective in helping to reduce or eliminate body odour. The precise mechanisms are not always known and much of the 'evidence' is based on individual reports rather than scientific evaluation. However, sufficient weight has been given to these anecdotal reports for many nutritionists to use the methods suggested below with a great deal of success.

The prestigious American publication *Prevention* has reported a number of anecdotes provided by its readers.

A Pennsylvania man . . . ended a long battle with body odour (which no deodorant would control) by taking 30 mg of zinc each day. He had no expectation that zinc would do this – he took it only because he felt that zinc would help his general health. Two weeks later he wrote that his body odour was gone.

Not improved but *gone*.

Another reader wrote, 'I had been troubled with underarm perspiration and odour and with perspiring feet.' Dusting powders failed to help him and underarm deodorants gave him a rash. After starting zinc supplementation he reported, 'I have no underarm odour, and my feet stay dry all day.'

Among the long list of conditions associated with zinc deficiency (in fact there are around 70 conditions and diseases listed) described in their book *The Zinc Factor*, authors Judy Graham and Dr Michel Odent include body odour. Why should we be low in this important trace element mineral?

Among the factors that reduce zinc levels are pregnancy, use of steroid medication such as cortisone, smoking and the contraceptive pill. You get zinc in your diet from oysters (between 45 and 70 milligrams of zinc per 100 grams of the food), liver (7.8 mg), shrimps (5.3 mg), cheese (around 4 mg), sardines (3 mg), wholemeal bread (2 mg) and eggs (1.8 mg). Also rich in zinc are sunflower and pumpkin seeds. Studies show that most people in industrialised countries do not eat enough zinc-rich foods and many are deficient. Most of us need around 15 milligrams daily, with breast-feeding women requiring more (25 mg).

Even if the diet is adequately supplying zinc, deficiency can occur because of poor absorption and use in the body due to other nutrient imbalances, most notably vitamin B6 and vitamin C. Additionally, several researchers have shown that under specific stress conditions – such as a sense of deep hopelessness – we produce excessive levels of a chemical called cortisol which blocks zinc function in the body. This condition, along with various hormonal imbalances, diabetes, increased levels of lead toxicity, and a diet that has excessive levels of saturated fats, all interfere with the way zinc functions, even if you are getting enough.

How can you know for sure whether you are zinc deficient? A test from a doctor can indicate levels but there are home methods that are quite accurate. One relies on the fact that when zinc is low we lose our sense of taste and smell to some extent – and sometimes completely. It is now possible to purchase from better health stores and nutritional supply companies a 'Zinc taste test' kit which provides you with liquid zinc. You place some in your mouth and if after 10 seconds you cannot register its distinctive taste you are very deficient. If after a few seconds you can taste something but not strongly then you are moderately deficient. If you pick up a strong taste immediately but don't find it unpleasant you are slightly deficient. If you taste something strongly and find it unpleasant you are fine and do not need extra zinc.

A second home test is to look at your finger nails – do they have lots of white flecks? If so you may well be zinc deficient.

If either of these tests are positive and you have B.O. you should try taking zinc (30 mg), vitamin C (1 gram) and B6 (100 mg) daily with meals for a few months, as well as following the general dietary advice given above.

CHAPTER NINE

Natural Help for the Hormones

We have seen that increased sweating is more common at puberty, when the feet tend to sweat more, and at the menopause, when it is hormonally linked to flushes. Interestingly these are also the times when zinc deficiency is more likely to occur or when zinc is more plentifully required.

The use of the Pill and other steroid (hormone-based) medications disturbs the metabolism and nutrient balance, especially of zinc and vitamin B6. The use of these drugs may be a major part of the cause of B.O. in some people. Low blood sugar, which can be a feature of B.O., is often related to excessive production of the hormone adrenaline, which stimulates sugar production as well as the heat centre of the brain, making us sweat more. We have already looked carefully at ways of normalising a hypoglycaemic condition. And if the thyroid gland is overactive it will certainly increase sweating.

So in a number of ways our hormones are linked to the level at which we sweat, as is the nervous system and its balance (see chapter 4). In previous chapters we have looked at ways of helping the imbalances of toxicity and deficiency that can be so involved in puberty-related and general health problems, using detoxification, supplementation and sound nutrition programmes. In this chapter we will briefly consider two other hormonal problems – menopausal hot flushes and overactive thyroid problems.

HOT FLUSHES

If there are menopausal problems related to excessive sweating the advice of a skilled nutritionist, herbalist or naturopath should be obtained, as there is much that can be done to help without using drugs. To help yourself, all the detoxification advice given earlier should be applied along with supplementation of vitamin E (600IU daily in three divided doses of 200IU each with meals) and selenium (200 microgrammes daily) and vitamin C (up to three grams daily with food). Use of these nutrients supplementally has had a positive effect in reducing sweating in menopausal women in many medical trials.

In addition it is often found that women suffering hot flushes have a great deal of muscular tension, especially in the neck and shoulder region, which can lead to local 'trigger point' formation – painful nodules which when pressed produce pain elsewhere. Regular massage and soft tissue manipulation can normalise the muscular condition and has been shown to be effective in reducing hot flushes dramatically. Such methods are more effective if combined with exercise – especially yoga type stretching – and relaxation methods such as those described in chapter 4.

OVERACTIVE THYROID

Take your early morning (before getting up) underarm temperature on three days running for a full 10 minutes. Find the average temperature by adding the three figures together and dividing by three. If the answer comes to above 98.2°F (36.8°C) then you probably have an overactive thyroid gland which could be causing excessive sweating.

If you also have a tendency to being thin and find it hard to gain weight, suffer insomnia, are highly emotional, have a tendency for your heart to race when you are resting, have night sweats and are disturbed by heat, preferring it cool, then the chances are very high that your thyroid is overactive. Tests of thyroid hormone levels in the bloodstream are less accurate than this simple do-it-yourself approach, which was developed by Dr Broda Barnes in the USA.

What can you do to reduce thyroid activity? It is

worth trying to follow the detoxification advice given in chapter 6 for several months and then rechecking the early morning temperature – it may have normalised, as toxicity is a major cause of thyroid imbalance. At the same time apply the stress-reducing breathing and relaxation methods described in chapter 4 (as stress affects the thyroid), along with some of the water therapy approaches to detoxification and relaxation suggested in chapter 6.

At the same time take the following supplements for two months and then recheck the thyroid activity by looking at your symptoms and early morning temperature:

Vitamin A – 10,000IU daily

Vitmain B complex (a high dosage formula containing not less than 50 mg of each of the major B vitamins) – one daily

Calcium citrate – 1000 mg daily

Potassium orotate – 1000 mg daily

Kelp (seaweed) – three tablets daily

Vitamin C – 3 grams daily

Eat a lot of the brassica family of foods – broccoli, cabbage, Brussels sprouts, cauliflower, kale – as well as mustard greens, soya beans, spinach, peaches and pears, as these can all reduce thyroid activity.

CHAPTER TEN

Design a Healthy Environment

Since most of us spend a great deal of our time indoors, at home or at work, it makes sense to try to create in those environments atmospheres that allow us to function at our best. We can also try to ensure that undesirable conditions, likely to increase the chances of body odour developing, are minimised. Clean healthy air, at an optimum temperature, can make us feel a good deal more energetic and can also prevent undue sweating and therefore body odour.

TEMPERATURE

Most modern homes and offices are too hot. Research has shown that physical work is performed most efficiently when the temperature is around 68°F (20°C). When temperatures reach 75°F (24°C) there is a reduction of about 15 per cent in the efficiency of work performed – and a lot more sweating. Where mental work is involved, 61°F (16°C) is the temperature that allows the work to be most efficiently performed without undue stress.

These temperatures may seem excessively low – and indeed might be too low for comfortable living and working for many people – but they should be kept in mind and compared with the temperatures in which you are working and living. Some compromise, in which temperatures are brought closer to these 'ideals', might be possible if changes towards a lower level of heating were made slowly – and this would certainly cut down sweating to some extent.

VENTILATION

Air movement also has a profound effect on how pleasant or unpleasant a work-space can be – and where double glazing and central heating coexist, lack of air movement can be a problem. Because of modern building design, in which rooms are virtually sealed boxes, it is not always possible to do much about having windows open, so fans might be needed to keep the air moving, even if this is only gently. If this is not possible it is a good idea to get outside for a few minutes several times a day for access to daylight and fresh air – even if that air is somewhat polluted.

IONISATION

Compounding the problem can be the excessive presence of positive ions in the air. Ions are electrically charged particles that enter our skin and lungs via the air around us. Positive ions which are negative in their effect on us, are produced by machinery and modern synthetic materials, and are also plentifully present in cigarette smoke.

To feel at our best the air we breathe is supposed to have a particular ratio (12:10) of negative to positive ions. We tend to feel fresher and more alert when ionisation is in this slightly negative balance.

In modern buildings, however, an imbalance is common in which there are usually far more positive ions than negative ones. A simple solution can be the installation, in offices, workplace or home, of an ioniser. These relatively cheap machines can make a huge difference, producing a feeling of freshness and alertness as they pump out negative ions into the atmosphere.

HUMIDITY

If humidity is extremely low, as is common where double glazing and mechanical heating are used, then a wide range of unpleasant physical effects, including problems related to sweating, are likely. When we are in an atmosphere where excessive humidity and heat coexist we tend to sweat more profusely, with the sweat staying on the surface of the skin. However, when humidity is extremely low, for example because of central heating which dries out the air, we may still sweat profusely when working (just as though we were in a sauna – where humidity is also very low) but we won't notice it as much because in these conditions the sweat has a greater chance to evaporate. Nevertheless some sweat residues stay on the skin and a good deal would find its way onto our underclothing; bacterial action would, after a couple of hours, start the process that leads to B.O.

The solutions to these problems demand that we create as healthy a working and living environment as possible. The following suggestions can make a dramatic improvement to your environment:

1 Try to ensure temperature control via use of thermostats so that the ambient temperature is kept at a level that encourages both efficiency and comfort but does not encourage lethargy and sweating – around 70°F (21°C) would seem ideal.
2 Have a fan strategically placed to keep the air moving if the room in which you work or where you spend most time at home is double or triple glazed, preventing windows from being opened. If windows can open then do so as frequently and as much as possible. Try to check that any heating system, whether solid fuel, gas or oil, has adequate and

efficient ventilation so that toxic fumes are not entering or remaining in the home or workplace.

3 Consider installing an ioniser near your place of work and/or at home. These small machines, about the size of a paperback book, simply plug into any electrical outlet and are silent and inconspicuous, as well as being inexpensive. They are especially needed in rooms where machines such as photocopiers, televisions and computer monitors are operating.

4 Whenever possible ensure that furnishings are made of natural materials in order to avoid exposure to the toxic chemicals that are released by most synthetic materials, many paints and varnishes, most wallpaper, modern synthetic carpeting and furniture, concrete and plastic. Try to obtain natural paper wall-coverings, wool, cotton or silk for carpets, furnishings and curtains, non-toxic wood, and clay, slate or ceramic materials.

5 Install humidifiers if there is central heating or air conditioning that is drying the air too much. Check that filters on air conditioning are adequate and clean.

6 Have as many green plants in rooms as you can, as these both increase humidity and clean the air of toxic gases such as carbon dioxide and formaldehyde, which is so prevalent in modern materials and buildings.

Access to fresh air and as much of it as possible, with real care over avoiding the negative elements described above, are major aids in reducing the effects of what has come to be known as 'sick-building syndrome'. The main ingredients of healthy air in the workplace are efficient, well-serviced, non-polluting machines for control of air quality, and the same applies to the home environment.

Resources

Most good health stores and many pharmacies will stock some of the specialised products listed and recommended in the various areas of the book focusing on particular health problems – such as vitamins, minerals, garlic capsules, and so on. Some products are imported and are not widely distributed. These are best obtained from their UK agents. For example Natren probiotic products ('friendly bacteria' such as *Lacidophilus*, *L.Bulgaricus* and *Bifidobacteria*) can be obtained from NutriWest, Buxton Road, New Mills, Stockport, Cheshire SK12 3JU (phone 0663-742753).

Natren and most health products (including essential oils, homoeopathic remedies, herbs, nutrients and 'crystal' deodorant stones) mentioned in this book can also be obtained from many health stores and specialist nutrient suppliers such as The Nutri Centre, 7 Park Crescent, London W1N 3HE (071-436-5122).

Clay products such as French clay soap and liquid soap can be obtained from the importers Kenbar Beauty Products, 20 Island Farm Avenue, Molesley Trading Estate, West Molesley, Surrey KT8 2UZ (081-979-7261).

Austrian (Neydharting) Moor products are available from White Ladies, Maresfield, East Sussex TN22 2HH (0825-762658).

Israeli Dead Sea Products can be obtained from Finders, Winchet Hill, Goudhurst, Kent TN18 1JY (0580-212062).

Weleda homoeopathic products are available by telephone from Weleda (UK) Ltd on 0602-309319, which is also a Helpline for those who would like basic information on the use of this approach.

Aromatherapy oils are now widely available at pharmacies and health stores as well as Body Shop outlets who also sell a number of other products discussed in the text such as specialised bath-mitts, natural bristle brushes and loofahs as well as non-chemical deodorants.

Caprylic acid (Mycopryl) antifungal tablets as discussed in relation to Candida treatment are available from BioCare, 54 Northfield Road, Kings Norton, Birmingham B30 1JH (021-433-3727). This company also supplies an excellent acidophilus and bifidobacteria product.

Linseed suggested for bowel health should be clearly manufactured for human consumption. A German brand Linusit – avilable from most health stores – is recommended.

Index